MALE CONTRACEPTIVES

The Modern Man's Easy Guide

Joshua John

TABLE OF CONTENTS

ABSTRACT

A pregnancy that wasn't planned is a worldwide public health issue. Although there is a wide selection of birth control methods for women, men have just the condom and vasectomy to choose from. Although surgical vasectomy can be undone in certain cases, condoms have a far lower success rate.

New forms of male contraception are desperately wanted and needed all over the world. Androgen plus progestin combinations show promise as a commercially viable, reversible male contraception during the next decade, and hormonal approaches have made the most progress in clinical development.

Researchers have shown the short-term safety and reversibility of hormonal male contraception by testing androgen plus progestin techniques employing oral, transdermal, subdermal, and injectable medication formulations. Weight gain, acne, mild reduction of serum high-density cholesterol, mood changes, and libido changes are the most often reported adverse effects of hormonal male contraception.

Hormonal male contraceptives have been shown to have higher contraceptive effectiveness rates than condoms in clinical studies. Little progress has been made in the development of non-hormonal male contraceptives; nonetheless, possibly reversible vaso-occlusive approaches are now under clinical studies in several countries.

Much research has shown that men and women alike want innovative male contraceptives. Lack of pharmaceutical company funding, worries about side effects and spermatogenic rebound associated with hormonal approaches, and a lack of unambiguous reversibility and demonstrated the efficacy of non-hormonal approaches are all factors slowing down research.

The eventual availability of male contraceptives will be a step towards reproductive justice and more fairness in family planning, and it has the potential to significantly reduce the number of unplanned births worldwide (now 40% of all pregnancies).

INTRODUCTION

Globally, there is a pressing need to reduce the prevalence of unwanted births. More than half of all unplanned pregnancies end in abortion, and this number is believed to be as high as 44% worldwide.

This increases the probability of dangerous medical treatments and potential maternal mortality for women. Despite several methods of birth control for women, these patterns remain, with millions of women having abortions in dangerous settings every year.

The majority of women who have an unwanted pregnancy are not using contraception or are not utilizing an effective technique, according to a new report by the World Health Organization (WHO) (e.g. withdrawal or the rhythm method). Discontinuing birth control due to health concerns, unwanted side effects, or a failed birth control attempt was a common occurrence.

When a woman stops using contraception for any of the aforementioned reasons, her partner may have few reversible options for preventing pregnancy. Two methods of birth control for men are now on the market: condoms and vasectomies.

The failure rate of condoms is 13%, even with consistent usage, while vasectomies are invasive and not always reversible. There is a lack of highly effective and reversible male contraception choices although research into developing these options is continuing.

Innovative techniques of male contraception are gaining attention from both men and women. Men are more likely than women to agree that both couples are equally responsible for family planning (78%). For couples when the female partner is unable to utilize female contraception owing to medical contraindications or side effects, a new male contraceptive would be a welcome alternative.

More than 60 years have passed since scientists first started investigating methods of male contraception, and in that time, we've come a long way. Here, we take stock of what has been accomplished in the realm of male contraceptive research and development, the obstacles that remain, the most promising studies yet, and what the future may hold.

CHAPTER 1

MECHANISMS OF MALE CONCEPTION

To prevent spermatogenesis from developing, hormonal male contraception interferes with the hypothalamic-pituitary-gonadal (HPG) axis, a naturally occurring hormonal feedback loop. The hypothalamus, which produces follicle-stimulating hormone and gonadotropin-releasing hormone, is the first step in a well-functioning HPG axis (GnRH).

In turn, this triggers the pituitary gland to secrete follicle-stimulating hormone and luteinizing hormone (LH) (FSH). Supporting the development of spermatogonia in the testes is the job of the Sertoli cells, which are helped along by FSH.

The production of testosterone by the testes is prompted by the luteinizing hormone (LH). Normal spermatogenesis requires an intratesticular testosterone concentration around 100-fold higher than that seen in blood. The feedback loop is completed by circulating testosterone, which blocks the production of GnRH, LH, and FSH.

The intrusion of hormones into male reproductive systems disrupts the HPG axis. Intratesticular testosterone synthesis and spermatogenesis are both suppressed by exogenous testosterone, whether taken alone or in combination with progestin. When combined with testosterone, progestins have direct inhibitory effects on the testes, which may enhance the rate and depth to which FSH and LH release suppression occurs.

While the amount of testosterone produced by the testicles is decreased, the exogenous androgen in the male contraceptive still attaches to androgen receptors in the brain and non-gonadal, peripheral tissues, allowing the man to keep his muscle mass and libido. The lack of sperm in the ejaculate is a reversible and, in many cases, a permanent side effect of suppressed spermatogenesis.

Male contraceptives that don't rely on hormones may do things like affect sperm motility or stop sperm from maturing in the testicles (intestinal).

Male Contraceptive Hormones

Several injectable formulations, transdermal gels, implants, and oral formulations have all been tested in clinical studies of male contraceptives.

Testosterone-Based Contraceptive Effectiveness Trials

"Efficacy studies" of contraception are clinical trials in which participants use the study technique exclusively. For the experimental drug to advance to this phase of research, it must first be proven to be safe for long-term treatment in males, all while achieving maximum suppression of FSH and LH.

Also, for the hormonal approach to function as a contraceptive, sperm production must be reduced to an unacceptable level. The average number of sperm in a milliliter of ejaculate from a healthy man is between 1 and 20 million. Data from early research on the effectiveness of male contraception showed that seamlessness (azoospermia) was not necessary for its effectiveness.

Effective male contraception is compatible with "severe oligozoospermia," defined as less than one million sperm per milliliter of ejaculate, with success rates comparable to those of female oral contraceptives.

Research on the effectiveness of male contraceptives is conducted in a way that minimizes the potential for unwanted pregnancies. Couples who sign up for the study must first go through a "suppression phase" in which they take other forms of birth control with the experimental product until the man's sperm count reaches a certain level (typically 1 million sperm/ml in the ejaculate).

This allows the pair to enter the study's "efficacy phase," during which they use just the experimental medicine as contraception while sperm concentration is monitored.

The first two studies on the effectiveness of hormonal male contraception were conducted by

WHO(World Health Organisation). Both trials had men inject 200 milligrams of testosterone enanthate (TE) into a muscle monthly, which is double the amount needed for natural testosterone replacement.

In the first trial, 70% of men reached the azoospermia threshold needed to enter the efficacy phase, whereas, in the second study, 98% of men reached the severe oligozoospermia (3 million/mL) threshold needed to join the efficacy phase.

The failure rate for this regimen was quite low, at just 1.4%. Men with sperm counts below 1 million per milliliter had a pregnancy rate of 0.7 per 100 persons-years. As a result of these results, the field now uses a threshold objective of 1 million/mL to enter the contraceptive effectiveness phase of a study including hormonal male contraception.

Participants often reported androgenic side effects such as acne, weight gain, mood changes, libido shifts, and abnormal liver function tests among other AEs. Some people experienced pain at the injection site. Because of this, the protocol was generally rejected by its target audience.

Testosterone undecanoate (TU) is a longer-acting IM formulation that was designed to decrease injection frequency (to monthly injections instead of weekly). Of the males who participated in the two trials evaluating this treatment plan, 97% had their sperm count reduced to below 3 million/mL, and 95% had their sperm count reduced to below 1 million/mL.

These investigations highlighted the phenomena of spermatogenic rebound (when one's sperm count climbs over the threshold during the effectiveness phase), which was likely responsible for the few births detected despite the good contraceptive efficacy reported (failure rates of 1.1-2.3%). Identical androgenic negative effects were seen despite the simplified dose regimen.

Studies On The Effectiveness Of Testosterone-Progestin Combined Contraception

The inhibition of spermatogenesis may be improved, and the potential for unfavorable androgenic effects can be mitigated when progestin is combined with androgen. In the first trial to examine the combination's effectiveness as a male contraceptive, researchers used testosterone implants in conjunction with IM depot medroxyprogesterone acetate (progestin) injections once every three months.

Men in 94% of studies reduced their sperm count to below 1 million per milliliter. Implant extrusion rates of over 10% in preliminary trials as well as uneven pharmacokinetics among testosterone implants precluded further advancement, even though no pregnancies occurred and fewer androgenic effects were documented.

Recent research on the effectiveness of injectable TU in combination with norethisterone enanthate was conducted on a global scale (progestin).

Ninety-six percent of the males reduced their sperm counts to below 1 million per milliliter, with just around two percent experiencing a failure rate.

The usual adverse effects of androgens were seen in this research. Nevertheless, the trial was cut short owing to the potential for side consequences, including sadness and mood disorders in certain individuals, according to an independent safety committee. Despite the study's premature conclusion, 72% of participants reported satisfaction with the approach, and just 6% stopped using the strategy owing to adverse consequences.

Antagonists of GnRH

As GnRH antagonists reduce circulating FSH and LH levels in males, they may be useful as supplements to male contraceptives that rely on androgens and/or progestins. To make matters worse, most research on GnRH antagonists (such as the short peptides Nal-Glu and acyline) have indicated that they do not appreciably improve the spermatogenic suppression brought on by the androgen/progestin regimen.

Another drug, cetrorelix (in combination with 19-nortestosterone), produces azoospermia consistently but is unattractive since it requires daily subcutaneous injections. GnRH antagonists have seen a decline in the study, yet they might be useful additions to androgen-based male contraception approaches.

CHAPTER 2

RECENT ADVANCES IN MALE HORMONAL CONTRACEPTION

Several male respondents to surveys regarding male contraceptives indicated a preference for daily pills over injections or implants. Nevertheless, a safe and effective oral formulation of testosterone or a testosterone agonist has been difficult to find. Potential oral male contraceptives include the new androgens DMAU and 11-MNTDC.

Dimethandienone Undecanoate (DMAU)

A variety of studies are looking at DMAU's efficacy as a male contraceptive, both orally and intramuscularly. Dimethandrolone (DMA), the active substance generated from the pro-drug DMAU in vivo, is a possible single-agent hormonal male contraceptive since it binds to both androgen and progesterone receptors.

There have been three studies done on oral DMAU in males. Oral administration of DMAU is food-dependent, although daily dosages of 200–400 mg DMAU significantly decrease serum testosterone, FSH, and LH concentrations to levels commensurate with contraceptive effectiveness.

Although the majority of study participants did report some negative side effects, the androgenic efficacy of DMA was confirmed by the fact that oral DMAU was well tolerated despite a significant reduction in blood testosterone concentrations.

Although hepatotoxicity was not seen, some patients did experience unwanted weight gain, a rise in hematocrit, a drop in HDL cholesterol, and a minor decrease in sexual desire. The results of a 12-week trial on the effects of oral DMAU on spermatogenic suppression have recently been compiled.

If DMAU is successful in reducing sperm counts, it would be a major advance toward creating a once-daily "male pill." Longitudinal research is needed to determine whether or not DMAU is safe and acceptable, and whether or not the absorption rate can be maintained without a significant increase in food consumption.

11β-methyl-19-Nortestosterone-17β-Dodecyl Carbonate (11-βMNTDC)

11-βMNTDC is an oral male contraception that binds to androgen and progesterone receptors like DMAU. Early research in humans confirmed the results of the animal experiments, showing that it was best taken with meals for optimal absorption. A 28-day, daily-dosing trial with oral 11-βMNTDC suppressed serum testosterone, FSH, and LH to extremely low levels, supporting its contraceptive effectiveness.

Among drug-treated people, weight and LDL-cholesterol increased, hemoglobin and creatinine increased somewhat, and sexual desire and HDL cholesterol decreased. To maximize benefits and minimize negative effects, 11-βMNTDC trials are being extended. 11-βMNTDC is being evaluated for injection.

The 7α-Methyl-19-Nortestosterone (M.E.N.T)

Even among synthetic androgens, MENT stands out for its strong androgenic activity. Subcutaneous implantation of MENT decreased spermatogenesis in males, however, this effect was short-lived. This might be because of side effects from using a more potent hormone implant. No progress has been made in developing this agent.

Combining Testosterone With Nestorone Gel (NES-T)

An investigational transdermal formulation combining testosterone and the powerful progestin nestorone (progesterone acetate) is in the works. Nestorone is distinguished as a "pure progestin" due to its exclusive progestogenic properties, in contrast to other synthetic progestins which may also have androgenic, anti-androgenic, or glucocorticoid binding capabilities in addition to activating the progesterone receptor.

Almost 88% of males in 6-month research had their sperm counts reduced to below 1 million/mL when using a combination of testosterone and nestorone to decrease blood FSH, LH, and testosterone concentrations.

The effectiveness of a gel containing both testosterone and nestorone is being tested in a phase 2b clinical trial right now. Four hundred married pairs from seven different nations are needed for this international research.

After the male partner's sperm count has decreased to below 1 million/mL, he and his spouse enter the effectiveness phase and depend only on the testosterone plus nestorone gel contraception for 12 months. The time frame for results is 2022–2023. This is the first hormonal male contraceptive effectiveness research to include a location in sub-Saharan Africa, and the first self-administered male hormonal contraception to achieve efficacy testing.

CHAPTER 3

PROBLEMS PREVENTING THE PROGRESS OF HORMONAL METHODS OF MALE CONTRACEPTION

The Adverse Effects and the Safety over the Long Term

Clinical studies of hormonal male contraceptives have often been encouraging for significant adverse effects until very recently. Researchers found no evidence of major side effects or long-lasting metabolic derangements in clinical studies of male contraceptives.

Nonetheless, there is still some doubt regarding the safety of androgen usage over the long term. Hormonal methods of male contraception are often associated with changes in metabolism and biochemistry, such as little weight gain, decreased HDL-cholesterol, and elevated hematocrit and hemoglobin levels.

These irregularities may or may not occur depending on the dose, the presence or absence of androgens, and the progestin. Hemoglobin and hematocrit are less likely to rise with transdermal formulations, for example, than with injectable formulations.

Weight gain is enhanced by the addition of progestin to a testosterone-based approach, as compared to testosterone alone, and HDL-cholesterol is reduced more noticeably with oral androgen administration than with injectable or transdermal formulations.

These alterations were not linked to an increase in the risk of unfavorable health outcomes in the vast majority of male contraceptive effectiveness studies (such as blood clots or cardiovascular events). The long-term effects of using these drugs, however, are yet unclear.

For instance, even though mild weight gain is often reported in these studies, whether the weight gain is connected with changes in body composition, such as increases in lean vs fat mass, is not evident and may have consequences for longer-term metabolic risk.

The human body is unable to convert several of the newer androgens (DMAU, 11-βMNTDC) into an estrogen-like molecule. The potential long-term consequences of the consequent decreases in serum estrogen on bone mass and strength are not measurable in a shorter-term investigation.

The need of investigating the psychological and sexual risks associated with male hormonal contraceptives was recently emphasized in research. Concerns about negative effects, such as changes in mood and despair, led researchers to suspend this effectiveness trial.

One case of depression was determined to be likely related to the contraceptive agent, one suicide was determined to be unrelated (the subject was unable to cope with academic pressure), one case of intentional paracetamol overdose and one case of tachycardia with paroxysmal atrial fibrillation were determined to be possibly related.

Fourteen of the 20 men who dropped out of the research cited emotional changes as the primary reason (or one of many reasons) for their withdrawal. Due to the lack of a placebo group, it is difficult to draw firm conclusions on the sexual side effects of male hormonal contraceptives. Several studies have shown both increases and decreases in libido with the same formulation.

Women often report shifts in mood and libido when they start using female hormonal contraception, but the causes behind these changes are still up for debate. In particular, it is not yet known the negative consequences regulatory authorities and potential male contraceptive users would be prepared to tolerate in return for the positive results of the method.

Female contraceptive risks are considered with the risks of pregnancy by women. In contrast, men who choose to utilize male contraception are doing so to protect their partner(s) from the possibility of pregnancy and any adverse consequences that may be connected with using a contraceptive.

Rates of Suppression and Recovery: One of the drawbacks of hormonal male contraception is the length of time it takes for men to inhibit normal spermatogenesis and then regain it once it has been suppressed.

Hormonal techniques need at least two to three months of usage to decrease spermatogenesis and achieve their full contraceptive effectiveness, since spermatogenesis is a 72-day cycle (from initial mitotic event to fully developed sperm).

That's about how long it takes for a vasectomy to start working. The median period for spermatogenesis to completely recover after suppression is also 3.4 months. Both the period of suppression and the period of recovery of spermatogenesis in males are very variable.

Age, race, baseline sperm and/or LH serum concentrations, mode of hormone administration, and usage of progestin may all play a role in this variation. Because of the extended "on" and "off" times, these techniques may not be as popular among males as other forms of birth control. All male hormonal contraception treatments are entirely reversible, despite the long waiting periods.

Failure to Suppress Spermatogenesis: Throughout all of the hormonal contraception studies, around 5-10% of men continuously fail to adequately suppress spermatogenesis to 1 million/mL.

While the cause is unclear, some men may continue to have low-level spermatogenesis due to the presence of chronic intratesticular testosterone and/or FSH/LH. According to a meta-analysis of previous research, spermatogenesis suppression occurs more quickly and consistently in Asian men than in non-Asian males of European heritage.

The cause of this discrepancy is unclear at this time. It's plausible that the same processes at work in "non-responders" cause those variances. It has been speculated that testicular histomorphometry, T concentrations and metabolism, androgen receptor polymorphisms, and gonadotropin suppressibility could all have a role.

Spermatogenic Rebound: Around one to two percent of men in trials that evaluate the effectiveness of hormonal contraception exhibit a transient increase in their sperm concentration that falls outside of the threshold for the effectiveness of the contraceptive.

This phenomenon is known as spermatogenic rebound. When sperm rebound occurs, the sperm count usually drops back within the effective range. There is still no understanding of what causes sperm to bounce back. This is not likely a difficulty with adhering to the regimen, since it has been found even in trials using long-acting androgens.

In the same way, it's plausible that sustained levels of testosterone and/or FSH/LH contribute to this transient rebound of spermatogenesis. This obstacle may soon be less of a problem since new technology may make it possible for men to test their sperm concentrations at home to determine their viability.

In conclusion, when it comes to hormonal male contraception, a combined androgen/progestin regimen has been shown via considerable research to have a high likelihood of delivering high contraceptive effectiveness that is reversible. Efforts to improve administration simplicity and fine-tune the dosage at which the risk/benefit balance is optimal are continuing areas of study.

CHAPTER 4

MALE CONTRACEPTIVES THAT DON'T RELY ON HORMONES

Non-hormonal male contraceptives are designed to prevent hormonal shifts, which may reduce the risk of systemic adverse effects. Several non-hormonal alternatives have progressed to the preclinical stage, demonstrating safety and efficacy in rodent models.

Targets unique to sperm are challenging to discover and have not been successfully translated from animal studies to human clinical trials. Particularly difficult has been the problem of "off-target" consequences when trying to hit all of these different substances and pathways at once.

Non-hormonal molecules necessary for sperm maturation, suppression of specific sperm motility machinery, and blockage of sperm transport to the ejaculate by reversibly occluding the vas deferens are all under research.

Methods of Vaso-Occlusion

RISUG, or Reversible Inhibition of Sperm by Guidance, describes the following process. The only non-hormonal technique of male contraception to enter clinical studies is vaso-occlusive methods.

These techniques, in theory, work by creating a temporary physical obstruction in the vas deferens lumen, preventing sperm from passing through, then releasing them once dimethyl sulfoxide (DMSO) is introduced. Vaso-occlusive therapies include RISUG and Vasalgel, both of which are injected intravenously twice (one in each arm).

RISUG: This is a vas intraluminal injection that has been studied for about 30 years in India. To prevent sperm from passing through the vas deferens, RISUG uses styrene maleic anhydride (SMA) to temporarily clog the vas deferens, changing the local pH and, therefore, the sperm's morphology (resulting in disrupted fertilizing ability).

Early investigations have shown that RISUG successfully suppressed testosterone production for at least a year and induced azoospermia in all male subjects within 1-3 months after injection. Several males had scrotal enlargement, and this was the most often reported adverse effect. Not a single pregnancy was mentioned in any of these investigations.

Most recently, 139 men participated in a phase III effectiveness trial. During the trial's duration, 133 of the men saw significant reductions in sperm count, with 82.7% experiencing azoospermia within 1 month and 17.3% between 3-6 months. Six men who did not successfully decrease sperm production throughout the procedure experienced complications.

Throughout the 6-month follow-up period, there were no pregnancies. Temporary scrotal enlargement was noted by the majority of individuals again, and minor discomfort in the scrotum and genital area was reported by 48 people (36.2%). (which was resolved within 1 month).

While reversibility has been hypothesized for RISUG, human experiments have yet to show it. Studies in rats, rabbits, and non-human primates showed that the effects might be reversed. Both invasive (injecting DMSO with or without sodium bicarbonate) and noninvasive (a multimodal strategy of maneuvers) attempts for reversal have been made. Before RISUG may be regarded as a form of reversible contraception and not permanent sterilization, human trials showing complete recovery of fertility are necessary.

Vasalgel: Similar to RISUG, vassalage is a bilateral vas injection that blocks sperm's ability to enter the vas deferens. However, the chemical makeup of vassalage is somewhat different from that of RISUG. A component of SMA acid is that it resists hydrolysis in water.

The benefits of low manufacturing costs and durability are thereby enhanced. Vasalgel showed significant suppression of sperm in pre-clinical research, with all rabbits reaching 1 million/ml within a month.

Vasalgel was reversed in some rabbits by injecting them with sodium bicarbonate, and although the concentration of their sperm was normalized, some morphological and motility problems remained. As a result, there was legitimate cause for alarm regarding the future of sperm function.

Vasalgel was shown to effectively prevent conception for 2 years in research involving 16 rhesus monkeys. No attempt was made to assess reversibility. There has been no research done on Vasalgel in humans.

Alternatives to Hormonal Methods of Contraception for Men

Adjudin, a lonidamine derivative, was an early nonhormonal contender that was shown to disrupt the Sertoli cell spermatid connections and the Sertoli cell cytoskeleton, leading to spermatid loss.

While the substance was shown to temporarily decrease spermatogenesis in rats, it required modification because of the inflammation and atrophy it caused in the liver and skeletal muscles.

In a further experiment, adjudin was linked to a recombinant FSH mutant to increase the latter's organ selectivity and facilitate its delivery to the testes. There was some worry about high manufacturing costs, limited bioavailability, and the potential of producing anti-FSH autoantibodies, even though this reduced off-target effects.

In recent years, effective and reversible infertility in rats has been caused by combining low (subtherapeutic) doses of adjudin with the endogenously produced reversible blood-testis-barrier modulator F5-peptide. Increased bioavailability and decreased systemic toxicity were achieved with the use of the F5-peptide and adjudin, respectively. Hence, adjudin and similar medicines that target Sertoli cells continue to show promise in pre-clinical testing.

The EPPIN sperm surface protein is another possible non-hormonal contraceptive target.

Research in monkeys has shown that infertility may be artificially produced by administering antibodies against EPPIN, which reduces sperm motility.

Reversible suppression of normal sperm motility in macaques was seen 30 hours after infusion with the EPPIN-targeting drug EP055. EP055 has the potential to be an "on-demand" contraceptive in the future, but further research into its safety and effectiveness is needed before it is tested on humans. Vitamin A and its metabolites may also be useful targets for developing non-hormonal methods of male contraception.

The vitamin A metabolite retinoic acid controls the expression of genes vital to proper spermatogenesis by binding to retinoic acid receptors (RAR). Administration of RAR antagonists may decrease spermatogenesis, as shown by infertility in RAR-knockout and vitamin A-deficient mice.

In male rats, the pan-RAR-antagonist BMS-189452 caused complete infertility, although this was reversible; unfortunately, side effects included testicular degeneration and signs of liver damage. Further research halved the dosage and doubled the treatment time of BMS-189453, achieving 100% induced infertility in mice with complete recovery and no off-target effects.

If a more selective RAR antagonist can be created to block solely RAR- activity in the sperm generation pathway, this approach shows promise as a potential non-hormonal male contraceptive option in the future.

Taken orally, the chemical WIN 18,446 blocks the production of retinoic acid in the testes. More than 50 years ago, it was shown that the male contraceptive WIN 18,446 could efficiently and reversibly suppress spermatogenesis; however, when combined with alcohol, the drug caused significant adverse responses in males, including nausea, vomiting, and malaise (disulfiram reaction).

Aldehyde dehydrogenase 1A2 (ALDH1A2) was identified as a possible effective and specific target in the retinoic acid production pathway to target a new inhibitor and potential contraceptive, in an attempt to disentangle the disulfiram response from the contraceptive effects. To that end, research into creating a bioavailable and selective inhibitor of ALDH1A2 is under conducted.

Many more potential candidates for a non-hormonal male contraceptive drug are now undergoing preclinical testing. Two of them are HC-056456, an inhibitor of the calcium ion channel (CatSper), which inhibits hyperactivation of sperm, and JQ1, an inhibitor of bromodomain testis-specific protein, which is essential for chromatin remodeling during spermatogenesis.

While still in the proof-of-concept phase, these potential contraceptive targets show long-term promise as reversible, non-hormonal male methods of contraception. The specificity of these inhibitors for sperm/spermatogenesis in humans is unknown since, as of yet, none have progressed to clinical trials.

CHAPTER 5

THE EFFECTS AND THE GENERAL ACCEPTANCE

In most parts of the world, when asked about the potential benefits of using male contraceptives, the vast majority of males express a desire for and a willingness to accept new methods of male contraception.

The majority of women would feel comfortable trusting their male partners to take a contraceptive if the data showed that their partners would do so. Despite the extensive interest shown by these polls, it is difficult to evaluate the acceptability of male contraception since no techniques are now available.

Men who have taken part in contraceptive clinical studies provide the most relevant data on acceptance, although these results are likely to be slanted in favor of receptivity and acceptability. In clinical investigations, the vast majority of males who used injectable or transdermal methods indicated satisfaction and readiness to suggest contraception to others.

In the male contraceptive research that was cut short because of worries about mood changes, 83% of participants said they would take similar hormonal contraception despite the risks if it were accessible.

The possible effects of male contraception on a global scale were modeled in recent research. The findings suggested that male contraception might lower the rate of unplanned births by 3.5-5.5% in the United States and by >30% in underdeveloped countries.

According to the findings, male contraception has the greatest potential to minimize unwanted pregnancies in areas where the usage of current contraceptives is low. Particularly in poor and underprivileged groups, where the implications of unwanted births may be the largest, it may be important to examine the effects of male contraception.

The pharmaceutical industry may be interested in speeding up the development of male contraceptives to market if more information is collected on the potential effect and acceptance of male contraception. The National Institutes of Health (NIH) is the primary funder of scientific research now (Eunice Kennedy Shriver National Institute of Child Health and Human Development).

Given the uncertain regulatory road to the clearance of a new agent, financial considerations are likely at the root of any decision to end funding. Yet, if forthcoming medicines show effectiveness, safety, and reversibility, worldwide opinions about male contraception and gender equality may shift over time, altering the current state of affairs.

CONCLUSION

New forms of male contraception are of interest and necessity all around the world. The perfect male contraceptive would have all the benefits of other methods while also being easy to use, non-invasive, and reversible. Male contraception might provide couples with an extra method of family planning and help bring the global rate of unwanted births down.

Several combinations of androgens and progestins, as well as androgens alone, have been studied for their effectiveness in male hormonal contraception. Androgen plus progestin regimens administered by injections and transdermal gels are now the most promising hormonal therapy, although new oral medicines are also being studied.

Clinical research results suggest these approaches are temporarily safe, reversible, and more effective than condoms for the vast majority of males. The hunt for a treatment plan that has minimal adverse effects is continuing.

Determining long-term safety, limiting and detecting "non-responders," and shortening the time it takes for a regimen to be successful and reversible are some more factors to think about.

Vaso-occlusive techniques have been the focus of most studies evaluating the efficacy of nonhormonal therapies, and further study is needed to validate their safety and reversibility. Numerous potential non-hormonal contraceptive targets are currently in the preclinical stages of research.

The introduction of innovative male contraceptives into the family planning market has been shown to have a high level of acceptance and the potential for beneficial effects. Reversible, safe male contraceptives are an important step toward reproductive equity because they allow men to take more active roles in family planning decisions.

MOST RELATED QUERIES

What is male contraception?

Male methods of contraception include vasectomy, withdrawal, and condom use. As a barrier method of contraception, condoms serve to prevent pregnancy because they stop sperm from reaching the uterus. The vas deferens, or sperm tubes, are permanently sealed up, obstructed, or severed during a vasectomy, making male contraception impossible. Withdrawal, or the pull-out procedure, is used when the male partner withdraws his vaginal clitoris from the female clitoris before ejaculating.

Male birth control surgery?

A vasectomy, the medical term for male sterilization, is a permanent method of contraception for males. The vas deferens, the tubes that transport sperm from the testicles to the urethra, are knotted, severed or sealed during the process. This method of birth control has a high rate of effectiveness and requires nothing in the way of preparation or recovery time.

New male contraceptive pill?

No commercially viable male contraception pill currently exists. But, scientists are working on a male contraceptive pill that would inhibit sperm creation by lowering testosterone levels and other relevant chemicals.

Male birth control trials?

Trials for male birth control are still being conducted, with some in the very early phases of clinical testing. Gels containing hormones, topical lotions, and implants are some of the most promising options. These hormone-infused gels and lotions effectively stop sperm production and stop sperm from being released after ejaculation. Hormones from the implants, which are placed in the scrotum, prevent the generation and motility of sperm. Other approaches, such as oral contraceptives and injectables that don't use hormones, are also in the research phase.

New male birth control?

Birth control methods for males are still in the early stages of development. Today's men may choose between condoms, vasectomy, and hormonal methods like testosterone and progestin for birth control. A new injectable contraception termed RISUG (Reversible Inhibition of Sperm Under Guidance) is now undergoing clinical trials in India. This injection may be used momentarily and is reversible to prevent sperm from leaving the body.

Weill Cornell medicine?

New York City is home to Weill Cornell Medical, an academic medical facility affiliated with Cornell University. Weill Cornell Physician Organization, Weill Cornell Graduate School of Medical Sciences, and Weill Cornell Medical College have all been part of Weill Cornell Medicine since its inception in 1898. NewYork-Presbyterian Hospital is the state-designated tertiary care center and level 1 trauma center in New York City, and it is connected with Weill Cornell Medical.

Contraception reproduction?

Reproduction entails the bringing into existence of new life, while contraception refers to the use of measures to prevent pregnancy.

What does male birth control do?

Hormonal methods of contraception for men operate by preventing ejaculatory sperm release. This form of contraception is currently in its early stages of research and development and is not commercially accessible at this time.

Does male birth control exist?

Yes, a method of contraception that works for men is available. Condoms, vasectomy, and hormone implants are just a few of the options available.

Soluble adenylyl cyclase?

Catalyzing the transformation of ATP into cAMP, soluble adenylyl cyclase is an enzyme found in membranes. This enzyme is critical for intracellular signal transduction and participates in many other cellular functions. Soluble adenylyl cyclase has several functions in the body, including signal transmission, gene expression control, and cellular metabolism.

What is spermicide?

An effective method of contraception for men, spermicide works to stop conception. An egg is protected from being fertilized by straying sperm. The vagina may be treated with a spermicide, a chemical that is rubbed in just before sexual activity. It may be used in conjunction with other methods of contraception, such as condoms, or on its own.

Male birth control study canceled

Recently, a male birth control research scheduled to take place in the UK had to be scrapped owing to a shortage of participants. The goal of the research was to establish the viability and usefulness of a temporary method of male contraception.

University College London was responsible for carrying out the research, with support from the UK's National Institute for Health Research. The research started enrolling participants in June 2019, but because of a dearth of male participants, the process was halted.

When the trial was halted, the researchers had only enrolled 40 of the targeted 500 males aged 18 to 45. The researchers claimed that the belief that this method of birth control would have negative impacts on fertility or sexual performance was to blame for the poor recruitment rate.

Researchers also found that few people were familiar with or aware of male contraception's advantages. This could have contributed to the poor recruitment rate by decreasing awareness and education.

It is the goal of the researchers that similar studies will be done in the future despite the discontinuation of this particular one. They think more men will volunteer for the research if they learn about the possibilities of male contraception.

.

www.ingramcontent.com/pod-product-compliance
Lightning Source LLC
Chambersburg PA
CBHW071144220526
45467CB00015B/1839